© [KLEIN HOYLE] [2024]

All rights reserved.

No part of this book may be reproduced, distributed, or transmitted in any form or by any means, including photocopying, recording, or other electronic or mechanical methods, without the publisher's prior written permission, with the exception of brief quotations in critical reviews and certain other noncommercial uses permitted by copyright law.

Disclaimer

The content in this book is based on the author's expertise and comprehension of the topic. The author has no affiliation or link with any corporation, business, or person. This book is meant to give general information and educational material only, and it should not be interpreted as professional medical advice. Always seek the advice of a skilled healthcare expert if you have any queries about medical issues or treatments. The author and publisher expressly disclaim any responsibility resulting directly or indirectly from the use or use of the information included in this book.

Table of Contents

CHAPTER 1 7
- An Introduction To Endoscopic Sinus Surgery 7
- Understanding The Sinuses 7
- Overview Of Endoscopic Sinus Surgery............8
- Evolution Of Endoscopic Techniques 9
- Common Sinus Conditions Treated with Surgery 10

CHAPTER 2 13
- Anatomy Of Sinuses 13
- Structure And Function Of Sinuses 13
  - 1. Maxillary Sinuses: 13
  - 2. Frontal Sinuses: 13
  - 3. Ethmoid Sinuses:.................................14
- Nasal Anatomy..15
- Sinus Drainage Pathways.............................16
- Key Anatomical Landmarks For Surgery..........17
  - 2. Middle Turbinate: 18
  - 3. Ethmoid Bulla: 18

CHAPTER 3 21
- Indications And Preoperative Evaluation 21

Criteria For Surgery.................................21
Diagnostic Tools And Tests.........................22
Patient Evaluation Process 24
   • Medical History:..............................24
Risk And Benefit Assessment 25
   • Benefits: 25
   • Risk:..26

CHAPTER 4..29
Surgical Instruments And Equipment 29
Introduction To Endoscopic Instruments.............29
   Forceps and Scissors: 30
Navigation Systems 31
Imaging Techniques Used During Surgery 32
Maintenance And Sanitizing Of Equipment 34
   Cleaning:......................................34
   Disinfection: 34
   Documentation: 35

CHAPTER 5..37
Surgical Techniques And Procedures 37
Basic Principles Of Endoscopic Surgery 37
   1. Visualization and illumination: 37

2. Instrumentation: 37
3. Navigation: 38
4. Minimally Invasive Approach: 38
Different Approaches To Sinus Surgery 38
1. Maxillary Sinus Surgery: 38
2. Ethmoid Sinus Surgery: 39
3. Frontal Sinus Surgery: 39
4. Sphenoid Sinus Surgery: 39
Step-By-Step Guide For Common Procedures....40
1. Maxillary antrostomy: 40
2. Ethmoidectomy: 41
3. Frontal Sinuotomy: 42
4. Sphenoidotomy: 42
Management Of Complications 43
1. Bleeding: 43
2. Orbital complications: 44
3. Cerebrospinal Fluid (CSF) Leak: 44
4. Infection: 44
CHAPTER 6 47
Anesthesia And Patient Safety......................47

Different Types Of Anesthesia Used In Sinus Surgery 47
    General anesthesia 47
    Local Anesthesia and Sedation 48
    Choosing the Right Anesthesia 49

Preoperative Patient Preparation 50
    Medical Evaluation 50
    Pre-operative Instructions 50
    Smoking and Alcohol 51
    Preparing mentally and emotionally 51

Intraoperative Monitoring 52
    Monitor Vital Signs 52
    Anesthesia Depth Monitoring 52
    Airway Management 53
    Managing Anesthesia Complications 53

Post-Operative Care And Pain Management 54
    Recovery Room Monitoring 54
    Pain Management 54
    Addressing Common Postoperative Symptoms 55
    Follow-up appointments 55
    Long-Term Recovery and Care 56

CHAPTER 7 57
Post-Operative Care And Rehabilitation 57
Recovery Timeline 57
Immediate postoperative period (first week) ... 57
Weeks 2-4 58
One to three months 58
Long-Term Recovery 59
Wound Care Instructions: 59
Nasal Irrigation 59
Avoiding Nasal Trauma 60
Keeping Nasal Area Clean 60
Monitoring for signs of infection 61
Potential Complications And Management 61
Bleeding 61
Infection 62
Nasal obstruction 62
Changes in odor or taste 63
Rehabilitation Exercises And Follow-Up Visits . 63
Breathing exercises 63
Physical activity 64
Follow-up visits 64

    Long-Term Care 65
CHAPTER 8: 67
    Advancements In Endoscopic Sinus Surgery 67
    Emerging Technologies 67
        High Definition Endoscopy 67
        Image-guided Surgery (IGS) 67
        Powered Instruments 68
        Balloon Sinuplasty 69
    Innovative Surgical Techniques 69
        Draf Procedures 69
        Minimally Invasive Approaches 70
        Use of Biological Adjuncts 70
        Office-Based Procedures 71
    Future Directions For Sinus Surgery 71
        Robotics for Sinus Surgery 71
        Regenerative Medicine 72
        Augmented Reality (AR) 72
CHAPTER 9 75
    Patient Education And Communication 75
    Educating Patients On Their Condition 75

Communicating The Risks And Benefits Of Surgery 77
Addressing Patients' Concerns And Expectations 79
Resources For Ongoing Support And Information 81
CHAPTER 10 84
Lifestyle Changes And Long-Term Management 84
Importance Of Lifestyle Changes 84
Strategies To Prevent Sinus Issues 86
Long-Term Treatment Of Chronic Sinusitis 88
Integrative Approaches To Sinus Health 91
Conclusion 94
THE END 97

ABOUT THIS BOOK

"Complete Guide to Understanding Endoscopic Sinus Surgery" is an invaluable resource for both medical professionals and patients, providing detailed insights into the complexities of this critical surgical technique. As the title indicates, this book digs into the intricacies of endoscopic sinus surgery, delivering a wealth of information organized into 10 expertly prepared chapters.

The initial chapter introduces readers to the principles of endoscopic sinus surgery, emphasizing the importance of knowing sinus anatomy and the advancement of surgical methods. This core information prepares readers for a more in-depth investigation of the anatomical components outlined in Chapter 2, where they will get a thorough grasp of sinus anatomy, function, and important landmarks critical for surgical accuracy.

One of this book's merits is its focus on comprehensive preoperative examination, as described in Chapter 3. Readers will learn about surgical criteria, diagnostic tools, and the significance of risk-benefit analysis. Chapter 4 broadens this knowledge by describing the various surgical tools, equipment, and imaging modalities required for effective surgical results.

Chapter 5 goes beyond theory to give a practical reference to surgical methods and procedures, including a step-by-step approach and insights into complications treatment. The critical necessity of patient safety is highlighted in Chapter 6, which looks into anesthetic alternatives, preoperative preparations, and postoperative care procedures, providing a comprehensive approach to patient well-being throughout the surgical journey.

Chapter 7 focuses on postoperative care and rehabilitation, guiding readers through the recovery schedule, wound care, and possible complication treatment, encouraging a thorough awareness of the patient's path outside the operating room. Chapter 8 takes readers on a journey into the future of sinus surgery, covering new technology, creative procedures, and case stories demonstrating recent breakthroughs, underlining the field's dynamic character.

Recognizing the importance of patient education and communication, Chapter 9 offers vital insights into how to successfully communicate with patients, resolve issues, and provide them with options for continued assistance. Finally, Chapter 10 emphasizes the significance of lifestyle changes and long-term treatment measures, calling for a more comprehensive approach to sinus health than surgical surgery.

In essence, "Complete Guide to Understanding Endoscopic Sinus Surgery" goes beyond the scope of a textbook, functioning as a beacon of information and direction for both practitioners and patients navigating the difficult world of sinus surgery.

Its extensive coverage, fascinating story, and practical insights make it an invaluable resource in the field of otolaryngology and beyond.

CHAPTER 1

An Introduction To Endoscopic Sinus Surgery

Understanding The Sinuses

Before getting into the complexities of endoscopic sinus surgery, it's important to understand the sinuses themselves. These air-filled spaces are found inside the bones of the skull and are coated by mucous membranes. The sinuses produce mucus, which moistens the air we breathe, traps dust and other particles, and improves our sense of smell.

The human skull has four pairs of sinuses: frontal, ethmoid, sphenoid, and maxillary sinuses. Each of these sinuses has its specific position and function. For example, the frontal sinuses are placed above the eyes and help filter and humidify breathed air, while the maxillary sinuses are behind the cheekbones and assist discharge of mucus from the nasal canal.

However, when the sinuses become inflamed or obstructed due to allergies, infections, or structural abnormalities, they may cause severe discomfort and result in symptoms such as nasal congestion, face pain, and trouble breathing. When conservative therapies such as medicines fail to offer relief, endoscopic sinus surgery may be considered to reduce symptoms and enhance sinus function.

Overview Of Endoscopic Sinus Surgery

Endoscopic sinus surgery is a minimally invasive treatment that involves the use of an endoscope, which is a thin, flexible tube with a camera and light source attached. This enables surgeons to see within the sinuses and make precise procedures without the need for typical incisions or severe tissue damage.

The surgery is usually conducted under general anesthesia, with the endoscope inserted via the nostrils to reach the sinuses. Once inside, the surgeon may check for obstructions, remove sick tissue, and widen the sinuses' natural apertures to facilitate drainage and ventilation.

One of the primary benefits of endoscopic sinus surgery is its ability to target particular sections of the sinuses while maintaining the surrounding healthy tissue. This leads to speedier recovery periods, less postoperative discomfort, and less scarring than standard open surgical approaches.

Evolution Of Endoscopic Techniques

Endoscopic sinus surgery has progressed significantly since its start in the 1980s. Initially, the surgery was largely used to treat chronic sinusitis that did not respond to medicinal treatment. However, advances in technology and surgical procedures have broadened the scope of endoscopic sinus surgery to cover a variety of sinus-related disorders, including nasal polyps, sinus tumors, and fungal sinusitis.

One of the most important advances in endoscopic sinus surgery has been the advent of navigation devices, which give real-time imagery and precise guidance to assist surgeons in navigating the complex architecture of the sinuses more safely and successfully. Furthermore, advances in equipment, such as powered shavers and microdebriders, have enabled more complete removal of diseased tissue while reducing harm to adjacent tissues.

As a consequence of these developments, endoscopic sinus surgery has become the gold standard for treating a variety of sinus problems, providing patients with better results and a greater quality of life.

Common Sinus Conditions Treated with Surgery

Endoscopic sinus surgery is recommended for a range of sinus disorders that have not responded well to conservative therapy. Some of the most prevalent indications for surgery are:

- Chronic sinusitis refers to sinus irritation that persists for 12 weeks or more, despite medical treatment.

- Nasal polyps are non-cancerous growths that may cause nasal congestion, face pressure, and decreased sense of smell.

- Sinus tumors are abnormal growths in the sinuses that may be benign or malignant. They need surgical excision for diagnosis and therapy.

- Recurrent acute sinusitis refers to repeated bouts of acute sinusitis that do not respond to antibiotics or other conservative treatments.

- Structural problems, such as a deviated septum or nasal bone spurs, may block sinus drainage and lead to recurring infections.

Endoscopic sinus surgery may provide patients with considerable relief from their symptoms as well as better sinus function and general quality of life.

CHAPTER 2

Anatomy Of Sinuses

Structure And Function Of Sinuses

The human sinuses are a network of hollow spaces found inside the bones of the face and skull that surround the nasal cavity. The maxillary, frontal, ethmoid, and sphenoid sinuses are all filled with air. Each sinus has a unique position and form, but they are all coated with mucous membranes and connect to the nasal passageways.

1. Maxillary Sinuses: The biggest sinuses are located in the cheekbones. They perform an important function in humidifying the air we breathe, improving the resonance of our voices, and reducing the weight of the skull.

2. Frontal Sinuses: Located above the eyes in the forehead bone, the frontal sinuses aid in the resonance of the voice and assist in the moisturization of breathed air. They may vary widely in size and form among people.

3. Ethmoid Sinuses: A complicated collection of tiny air cells placed between the eyes. They are split into three groups: anterior, middle, and posterior, and they help to filter and humidify the air we breathe.

4. The sphenoid sinuses, located deep inside the skull beyond the nasal cavity, are critical for preserving the skull's structural integrity and providing a channel for nerves and blood vessels.

These sinuses have various roles, including reducing the weight of the skull, producing mucus that moisturizes the inside of the nose, trapping particles and infections, enhancing our voices, and serving as a buffer to protect essential components such as the eyes and brain.

Nasal Anatomy

Understanding the nasal anatomy is critical for understanding sinus surgery. The nasal septum divides the nose into two parts: exterior and interior, respectively. The exterior nose is composed of nasal bones and cartilage, while the internal nose comprises the nasal cavity, which is divided into two halves by the septum.

1. The nasal cavity runs from the nostrils to the back of the throat. It is lined with a mucous membrane that collects dust and bacteria. The nasal septum divides the nasal cavity into two nostrils, each containing superior, middle, and inferior nasal conchas (turbinates).

2. The nasal septum is a vertical wall that separates the nasal cavity into two sections. It is composed of bone and cartilage. Deviation or injury to the septum may cause breathing issues and need surgical intervention.

3. Turbinates are long, thin bone shelves that extend into the nasal cavity. They assist to warm and humidify the air we breathe. The turbinates are lined with mucous membranes and perform an important function in filtering breathed air.

Sinus Drainage Pathways

Each sinus has a unique drainage channel that permits mucus to discharge into the nasal cavity. Proper drainage is essential for avoiding sinus infections and maintaining good sinus health.

1. The maxillary sinuses drain into the middle meatus of the nasal cavity via the ostium. This route may become obstructed owing to inflammation or structural abnormalities, resulting in sinusitis.

2. The frontal sinuses drain into the middle meatus via the frontonasal duct. Blockage of this duct may cause frontal sinusitis, which causes headaches and pressure in the forehead.

3. Ethmoid Sinus Drainage: The anterior ethmoid cells empty into the middle meatus, whereas the posterior ethmoid cells exit into the superior meatus. Infections in this area may be very dangerous since they are so close to the eyes and brain.

4. Sphenoid Sinus Drainage: The sphenoid sinuses drain into the sphenoethmoidal recess, which is situated in the rear of the nasal cavity. Infections here may cause severe headaches and other neurological problems.

Key Anatomical Landmarks For Surgery

During endoscopic sinus surgery, physicians use precise anatomical markers to guide and conduct treatments safely. These markers help to avoid damage to important structures and ensure efficient therapy.

1. The uncinate process is a crescent-shaped bone protrusion in the lateral wall of the nasal cavity.

It is a critical marker for accessing the maxillary sinus ostium and ethmoid sinuses. The removal of this bone after surgery helps enhance nasal drainage.

2. Middle Turbinate: This structure is essential for determining the middle meatus and ethmoid infundibulum. The middle turbinate is often shifted or removed to increase sinus access and ventilation.

3. Ethmoid Bulla: A conspicuous air cell in the ethmoid bone, one of the first structures seen after ethmoid sinus surgery. Identifying and opening the bulla provides access to deeper ethmoid cells and the frontal sinus recess.

4. The sphenoid ostium, located in the sphenoethmoidal recess, is the entry of the sphenoid sinus. Identifying this ostium is critical for securely accessing and draining the sphenoid sinuses.

5. The orbit and lamina papyracea are the thin bones that separate the ethmoid sinuses from the orbit (eye socket).

Surgeons must explore this region with caution to avoid harming the eye and adjacent structures.

Understanding the anatomical landmarks and their interactions is essential for safe and successful endoscopic sinus surgery. Mastery of this anatomy enables surgeons may treat sinus problems without causing injury to other essential structures.

CHAPTER 3

Indications And Preoperative Evaluation

Criteria For Surgery

Endoscopic sinus surgery (ESS) is often used when patients have chronic sinusitis or other sinus-related diseases that do not respond well to conventional therapy. The factors for suggesting ESS are:

• Chronic rhinosinusitis (CRS) refers to sinus inflammation that persists for more than 12 weeks despite medical treatment such as antibiotics, nasal steroids, and saline irrigation.

• Recurrent Acute Rhinosinusitis refers to many bouts of acute sinusitis within years that need antibiotic therapy.

• Nasal polyps, which obstruct airflow and drainage, are typically linked to chronic rhinosinusitis.

- Fungal Sinusitis refers to invasive or allergic fungal infections that cause sinus obstructions and inflammation.

- Sinus tumors are benign or malignant growths that block the sinuses and need to be removed.

- Structural abnormalities, such as a deviated septum or concha bullosa, may cause sinus blockage.

- Surgical intervention may be required for sinusitis complications, such as orbital cellulitis, abscess, or intracranial problems.

Diagnostic Tools And Tests

Before surgery is contemplated, a thorough diagnostic assessment is required to confirm the diagnosis and discover the root causes of sinus problems. The key diagnostic tools and tests are:

- Nose endoscopy involves inserting a thin, flexible tube with a camera (endoscope) into the nose passages to see the sinus cavities and entrances.

This method allows for a thorough inspection of the nasal mucosa, including the detection of polyps and the identification of pus or mucus.

- High-resolution CT scans of the sinuses may detect anomalies such as polyps, tumors, or anatomical aberrations. It aids in the planning of surgical procedures.

- Magnetic Resonance Imaging (MRI) may be advised for soft tissue detail in situations of suspected malignancies or fungal sinusitis.

- Identifying and controlling allergies is critical for preventing persistent sinus irritation. Skin prick testing or specialized IgE blood tests are widely utilized.

- Swabs from nasal passages or sinuses may detect bacterial, fungal, or viral infections, directing antibiotic or antifungal treatment.

- Blood tests may be required to check for illnesses such as immunodeficiency or systemic inflammatory diseases that might impact sinus health.

Patient Evaluation Process

A complete patient examination is required to establish appropriateness for endoscopic sinus surgery and maximize results. The evaluation method includes:

- **Medical History:** Gather detailed information on the patient's symptoms, treatment history, response to therapy, allergies, asthma, and any pertinent illnesses.

- A thorough ENT examination focuses on the nasal cavities, throat, and ears. Nasal endoscopy is often used during this examination to get a direct view of the nasal passages.

- Use validated symptom ratings, such as the Sino-Nasal Outcome Test (SNOT-22), to assess the intensity of symptoms and their effect on quality of life.

- Review CT or MRI images for anatomical abnormalities, disease extent, and possible surgical intervention.

- Optimize medical management before surgery. This comprises antibiotics, nasal corticosteroids, saline irrigations, and maybe oral steroids or antifungal medicines.

- For difficult patients, visits with allergists, pulmonologists, or immunologists may be necessary to treat concomitant disorders such as asthma, cystic fibrosis, or immunological deficiencies.

Risk And Benefit Assessment

Understanding the risks and advantages of endoscopic sinus surgery is critical for informed consent and collaborative decision-making. Key points include:

- **Benefits:**
Symptom Relief: Improves nasal congestion, face discomfort, and pressure, and reduces sinus infections.

Improved Quality of Life: Improves sense of smell, sleep, and everyday functioning.

Reduced medication use, including antibiotics and nasal steroids.

Treatment of underlying conditions includes removing polyps, tumors, and fungal debris that do not respond to medicinal treatment.

- **Risk:**

Bleeding, although often minimal, may need extra attention.

Postoperative infections are infrequent but may need antibiotics.

The closeness of the sinuses to the eyes poses a slight risk of orbital damage, which may impair vision.

Cerebrospinal Fluid Leak: Because the sinuses are near the brain, there is a rare risk of cerebrospinal fluid leak, which may need further surgical intervention.

Risks of anesthesia include allergic responses and problems from underlying health disorders, similar to any other procedure.

By completely comprehending these features, patients may make educated choices about having endoscopic sinus surgery and predict the procedure's results and possible obstacles.

CHAPTER 4

Surgical Instruments And Equipment

Introduction To Endoscopic Instruments

Endoscopic sinus surgery necessitates the use of a variety of specialized devices that allow surgeons to maintain exact control and sight inside the nose passageways' tiny spaces. Endoscopes, forceps, suction devices, microdebriders, and other cutting and gripping tools are among the equipment used.

The major tool in endoscopic sinus surgery is the endoscope, which is a slim, tubular device containing a light source and a camera. Endoscopes are available in various diameters (usually 4mm for adults and 2.7mm for children) and angles (0, 30, 45, and 70 degrees) to offer distinct views of the nasal canal and sinuses. The kind of endoscope used depends on the region under examination or treatment.

Forceps and Scissors: Different kinds of forceps (such as Blakesley forceps) and scissors are used to grab and cut tissue. Blakesley forceps, for example, come in many shapes, including straight, upturned, and angled, enabling surgeons to access and manipulate tissues in limited areas.

Suction devices are vital for keeping the surgery field clean by removing blood and other fluids. They vary in size and form to accommodate various parts of the nasal cavity.

Microdebriders are powered tools with revolving blades that remove soft tissue and bone. They enable accurate and controlled tissue removal, lowering the danger of harming nearby structures.

Other specialized instruments include angled curettes for scraping and removing sick tissue, as well as frontal sinus searchers and dilators for entering and expanding sinus apertures.

Navigation Systems

Navigation systems are an essential component of contemporary endoscopic sinus surgery, offering real-time, three-dimensional guidance that improves accuracy and safety. These devices combine preoperative CT or MRI images with intraoperative data to assist surgeons with complicated sinus anatomy.

Navigation systems utilize electromagnetic or optical tracking to match the location of surgical tools to preoperative images. This enables surgeons to see the precise placement of their tools relative to the patient's anatomy in real-time on a monitor.

A navigation system's main components are a computer workstation, a tracking system (electromagnetic or optical), a reference frame coupled to the patient, and instrument-mounted sensors. To match the patient's anatomy with preoperative photographs, the system must be calibrated and registered initially.

Advantages: Navigation systems improve sinus surgery precision, particularly in situations with altered anatomy owing to prior procedures or illness. They enable surgeons to avoid crucial areas including the optic nerve and the brain, lowering the chance of problems. They are especially effective for revision procedures and difficult situations.

Imaging Techniques Used During Surgery

Endoscopic sinus surgery requires accurate imaging to plan and execute. Various imaging modalities give precise images of the nose and sinus architecture, which helps with diagnosis, surgical planning, and intraoperative guiding.

Computerized Tomography (CT) scans are the gold standard for preoperative evaluation in sinus surgery.

They give precise, high-resolution pictures of the sinuses' bony structures, highlighting disease severity and structural differences. CT scans are utilized to construct the 3D models used in navigation systems.

Magnetic Resonance Imaging (MRI): Although less typically utilized than CT for regular sinus surgery, MRI may be very useful for examining soft tissue structures, such as finding malignancies or inflammatory illnesses that extend into the orbit or brain. MRI is often used in concert with CT to offer a complete picture of the operative site.

Intraoperative Imaging: Some sophisticated surgical suites include intraoperative CT or cone beam CT (CBCT) scanners. These provide real-time imaging during surgery, ensuring that diseased tissue is precisely removed and sinus passageways are properly opened.

Maintenance And Sanitizing Of Equipment

Proper cleaning and maintenance of surgical instruments is crucial for avoiding infections while also guaranteeing the equipment's lifetime and usefulness. This includes rigorous cleaning, disinfecting, and regular maintenance procedures.

Cleaning: Instruments should be cleaned immediately after surgery to remove any blood, tissue, or debris. This usually entails physical cleaning with brushes and enzyme detergents to remove organic debris, followed by a rinse.

Disinfection: Once cleaned, instruments are disinfected using high-level disinfectants or automated washer-disinfectors. This process kills most harmful germs, but not all spores.

Sterilization is the ultimate phase, which eliminates all forms of microbiological life, including spores. Steam sterilization (autoclaving), ethylene oxide gas, hydrogen peroxide plasma, and peracetic acid sterilization are some of the most common procedures. The technique used is determined by the material and design of the instrument.

Regular maintenance is required to ensure that instruments stay in excellent operating order. This involves regular wear and damage inspections, blade sharpening, and adequate lubrication of moving components. Instruments should also be kept in a way that minimizes damage and contamination.

Documentation: Keeping thorough records of sterilization cycles and maintenance procedures is critical for ensuring compliance with healthcare laws and tracing the history of each equipment. This documentation assists in recognizing problems and maintaining a consistent quality of service.

Understanding the complexities of surgical equipment, navigation systems, imaging modalities, and sterilizing procedures may help healthcare practitioners ensure the effectiveness and safety of endoscopic sinus surgery.

CHAPTER 5

Surgical Techniques And Procedures

Basic Principles Of Endoscopic Surgery

Endoscopic sinus surgery (ESS) is a minimally invasive surgical method that aims to restore sinus airflow and function. The fundamental concepts of endoscopic surgery include using a nasal endoscope, and specialized equipment, and carefully navigating the complicated architecture of the sinus passages.

1. Visualization and illumination: The endoscope allows a good view of the nasal and sinus anatomy. It has a light source that illuminates the region, enabling the surgeon to see clearly and make accurate movements.

2. Instrumentation: Microdebriders and powered shavers are utilized to remove blockages and diseased tissue. These devices are intended to function inside the limited limitations of the nasal passageways.

3. Navigation: Advanced navigation systems may help improve the procedure's safety and precision. These devices provide real-time, three-dimensional imaging of the sinuses, allowing surgeons to avoid important tissues including the optic nerve and brain.

4. Minimally Invasive Approach: The objective is to minimize tissue injury while preserving as much native architecture as feasible. This method decreases surgical discomfort, accelerates healing, and minimizes complications.

Different Approaches To Sinus Surgery

There are various ways to sinus surgery, each customized to a particular problem or location of the sinuses. The technique used is determined by the patient's anatomy, illness severity, and surgical aims.

1. Maxillary Sinus Surgery: This method entails making an opening in the maxillary sinus, which is situated in the cheek.

The natural ostium (opening) of the maxillary sinus is expanded to promote drainage and ventilation. This treatment is often used to treat chronic maxillary sinusitis and remove polyps.

2. Ethmoid Sinus Surgery: The ethmoid sinuses are a complicated network of air cells that connect the eyes. Ethmoidectomy is the removal of damaged ethmoid air cells to improve sinus drainage. This treatment is often used to treat ethmoid sinusitis and polyps.

3. Frontal Sinus Surgery: Accessing the frontal sinuses, which are positioned in the forehead, may be difficult owing to their position. Frontal sinusotomy entails expanding the frontal sinus drainage route. This method is used to treat frontal sinusitis and remove blockages like polyps or mucoceles.

4. Sphenoid Sinus Surgery: The sphenoid sinuses are situated behind the nasal cavity and toward the base of the skull.

Sphenoidotomy is a procedure that opens the sphenoid sinus to increase drainage and cure problems such as sphenoid sinusitis or malignancies.

Step-By-Step Guide For Common Procedures

Understanding the step-by-step process of typical endoscopic sinus operations may help patients and healthcare providers better prepare for the procedures.

1. Maxillary antrostomy:

Preparation: Anesthetize the patient and decongest the nasal cavity using a vasoconstrictor.

The endoscope is introduced softly into the nasal cavity.

Identify key features, including the central turbinate and natural ostium of the maxillary sinus.

The antrostomy procedure involves widening the natural ostium using a microdebrider or powered shaver.

Debridement involves removing diseased tissue or polyps to improve sinus outflow.

2. Ethmoidectomy:

Preparation involves anesthetizing the patient and decongesting their nose.

The endoscope is inserted into the nasal cavity.

Landmarks identified include the central turbinate and the ethmoid bulla.

Diseased ethmoid air cells are carefully removed using precise equipment.

- Drainage Pathway Clearance: Inspect and clean nearby sinus drainage passages as needed.

3. Frontal Sinuotomy:

Preparation: Anesthesia and nasal decongestion are administered.

The endoscope is placed into the nasal cavity.

Landmarks highlighted include the middle turbinate and frontal recess.

Enlarging the frontal sinus drainage channel improves sinus ventilation.

Clear drainage is ensured by removing any obstacles, including polyps.

4. Sphenoidotomy:

Preparation: Anesthesia and nasal decongestion are administered.

The endoscope is placed into the nasal cavity.

Landmarks are recognized, including the sphenoethmoidal recess.

Sphenoid sinus opening involves enlarging the ostium.

Removal of obstructive tissue improves sinus outflow.

Management Of Complications

Endoscopic sinus surgery is precise and minimally invasive, yet problems may still occur. Effective care of these problems is critical to patient safety and excellent results.

1. Bleeding:

Intraoperative management involves controlling bleeding with hemostatic procedures including cauterization and packing.

Nasal packing or hemostatic medications may be used to manage postoperative bleeding. Patients should avoid activities that may raise blood pressure, such as heavy lifting.

2. Orbital complications:

To avoid orbital damage, it's important to navigate carefully and identify anatomical markers.

To manage an ocular problem such as a hematoma, visit an ophthalmologist right away.

3. Cerebrospinal Fluid (CSF) Leak:

To prevent skull base breaches, employ navigation systems and practice proper techniques.

Management: CSF leaks are treated intraoperatively using grafts or sealants. Bed rest and head elevation are common postoperative procedures.

4. Infection:

Sterile procedures and postoperative care may reduce the risk of infection.

Management: Antibiotics are used to treat infections. Serious cases may need surgical drainage.

5. Scar Formation and Adhesion:

To prevent scar development, apply anti-adhesion gels and handle tissues gently.

Adhesions are addressed with meticulous debridement during follow-up visits.

Understanding the ideas, techniques, stages, and treatment strategies in endoscopic sinus surgery allows healthcare providers and patients to be more prepared for the procedure and any difficulties, resulting in safer and more successful results.

CHAPTER 6

Anesthesia And Patient Safety

Different Types Of Anesthesia Used In Sinus Surgery

General anesthesia

General anesthesia is the most often utilized kind of anesthesia in endoscopic sinus surgery. It entails making the patient entirely unconscious and painless. This form of anesthesia keeps the patient calm and comfortable during the process, which is important given the delicate nature of sinus surgery. The technique usually starts with the injection of intravenous medicines to induce unconsciousness. Once the patient is sleeping, a breathing tube is put into the windpipe to keep the airway open and supply a combination of anesthetic gases and oxygen.

General anesthesia provides a regulated and predictable state of unconsciousness, full muscular relaxation, and control over the patient's respiration. This is especially crucial in sinus surgery when even little motions might cause complications. However, general anesthesia requires close monitoring by an anesthesiologist to treat possible adverse effects such as blood pressure and heart rate changes.

Local Anesthesia and Sedation

In rare circumstances, sinus surgery may be conducted with local anesthetic and sedation. This method includes numbing a particular region of the sinuses with a local anesthetic while simultaneously administering sedatives to help the patient relax and minimize anxiety. Sedation may vary from moderate, in which the patient is awake but relaxed, to severe sedation, in which the patient is on the edge of sleep but can still react to certain stimuli.

Local anesthesia with sedation is often recommended for small sinus operations or for individuals who have medical issues that make general anesthesia risky. This approach offers a faster recovery period and fewer side effects than general anesthesia. However, the patient must be agreeable and capable of keeping still during the procedure.

Choosing the Right Anesthesia

The kind of anesthetic used depends on various aspects, including the scope of the sinus surgery, the patient's general health, and personal preferences. During the preoperative consultation, the surgeon and anesthesiologist will review the available choices with the patient to identify the most suitable and safe anesthetic strategy.

Preoperative Patient Preparation

Medical Evaluation

Patients are evaluated thoroughly before having endoscopic sinus surgery to determine their general health and preparedness for anesthesia. This assessment usually involves a thorough medical history, a physical exam, and sometimes blood tests and imaging scans. Patients are questioned about any chronic illnesses, allergies, drugs, and past responses to anesthesia.

Pre-operative Instructions

Patients are given particular advice to prepare for surgery. To lessen the danger of aspiration under anesthesia, it is common to fast for some time before the surgery. Patients are frequently instructed to avoid eating and drinking at midnight the night before their procedure.

They may also be advised to cease certain drugs, such as blood thinners, which may raise the risk of bleeding.

Smoking and Alcohol

Patients who smoke are strongly advised to stop at least several weeks before surgery since it may hinder wound healing and increase the risk of complications. Similarly, in the days before surgery, alcohol use should be limited or avoided to lower the risk of anesthesia-related complications.

Preparing mentally and emotionally

Preoperative nervousness is common, and patients are encouraged to communicate their worries to the surgical team. Understanding the operation, anesthetic strategy, and anticipated results might assist in reducing anxiety. In rare situations, a moderate sedative may be used to assist the patient in resting the night before surgery.

Intraoperative Monitoring

Monitor Vital Signs

Endoscopic sinus surgery requires regular monitoring of the patient's vital signs to guarantee safety and handle any issues as soon as possible. The following vital indicators are monitored: heart rate, blood pressure, oxygen saturation, and respiration rate. This monitoring is carried out utilizing sophisticated technology that sends real-time data to the surgical and anesthetic teams.

Anesthesia Depth Monitoring

To maintain an optimum degree of anesthesia, the anesthesiologist uses a variety of techniques to monitor the depth of anesthesia. This might include clinical symptoms like pupil response, blood pressure, and heart rate, as well as sophisticated technologies like bispectral index (BIS) monitoring, which examines brain activity to determine the patient's state of awareness.

Airway Management

Proper airway control is crucial during general anesthesia. The anesthesiologist makes sure the breathing tube is properly inserted and monitors the patient's breathing during the treatment. In the case of local anesthesia sedation, oxygen replacement, and airway patency are constantly monitored.

Managing Anesthesia Complications

The anesthesia staff is prepared to handle any problems such as allergic responses, blood pressure abnormalities, and breathing concerns. A well-equipped operating room and competent staff guarantee that any concerns may be handled quickly and efficiently.

Post-Operative Care And Pain Management

Recovery Room Monitoring

After the procedure, the patient is sent to a recovery room and carefully observed while they awaken from anesthesia. Vital signs are continuously checked, and the patient is evaluated for any acute postoperative complications such as nausea, vomiting, or breathing problems. During this important phase, nurses and anesthesiologists give care and support.

Pain Management

Effective pain management is an essential component of postoperative treatment. Pain drugs are often administered to patients to alleviate their agony. Non-steroidal anti-inflammatory medications (NSAIDs) for mild to moderate pain and opioids for severe pain are possible options.

In certain circumstances, localized pain management methods, such as nerve blocks or topical anesthetics, may be employed.

Addressing Common Postoperative Symptoms

It is usual for people to have nasal congestion, slight bleeding, and pain after sinus surgery. Instructions for managing these symptoms, such as using saline nasal sprays, humidifiers, and elevating the head, are offered. Patients should avoid vigorous activity and adhere to certain post-surgery protocols to facilitate recovery.

Follow-up appointments

Follow-up consultations are necessary to check the patient's healing progress. During these visits, the surgeon checks the surgery site, removes any packing or splints, and answers any questions the patient may have. Follow-up care ensures that issues are detected and treated as soon as possible.

Long-Term Recovery and Care

Endoscopic sinus surgery might need several weeks to fully recuperate. Patients are given extensive instructions on wound care, medication use, and symptoms of possible problems to look out for. Maintaining proper nose hygiene and attending all follow-up consultations are essential for getting the greatest results.

Patients may approach endoscopic sinus surgery with confidence if they understand the anesthetic procedure, preoperative preparation, intraoperative monitoring, and postoperative care. This ensures that their safety and comfort are emphasized throughout the surgical journey.

CHAPTER 7

Post-Operative Care And Rehabilitation

Recovery Timeline

The recovery period after endoscopic sinus surgery is essential, requiring close monitoring and attention to postoperative care guidelines. Understanding this timeframe allows patients to have reasonable expectations and ensures they are appropriately prepared for the recovery process.

Immediate postoperative period (first week)

Patients often feel nasal congestion, mild bleeding, and pain in the days immediately after surgery. During this time, you must strictly adhere to the surgeon's directions. Patients may feel exhausted and should rest as much as possible. Using saline nasal sprays as advised keeps the nasal passages wet and aids recovery.

Pain is normally treated with prescription medicines, and antibiotics may be used to avoid infection.

Weeks 2-4

As the edema and irritation lessen, individuals may still have nasal obstruction and discharge. During this period, saline nasal rinses should be used regularly to help clean up mucus and crusts. During this time, follow-up visits are typical to allow the surgeon to inspect the nasal passageways and remove any crusts or debris that may impede recovery.

One to three months

Most people feel much better after the first month. The nasal passages continue to heal, and breathing via the nose gradually improves. Follow-up visits are crucial for monitoring development and addressing any developing concerns. During this time, patients may be permitted to resume regular activities, but they should avoid intense activity or activities that might cause nasal injury.

Long-Term Recovery

Complete recovery and the outcome of the procedure might take many months. Patients should continue with nasal irrigation and follow any special recommendations from their healthcare practitioner. Regular follow-up sessions are required to ensure that the sinuses heal correctly and to address any long-term issues that may develop.

Wound Care Instructions:

Proper wound care is critical for preventing infection and promoting healing after endoscopic sinus surgery. Here are explicit instructions for patients to follow:

Nasal Irrigation
Regular nasal irrigation is an essential part of wound care. Patients should flush their nasal passages with saline several times each day to keep them clean and

moist. This helps to wash out mucus, blood clots, and debris, lowering the risk of infection and speeding up recovery. A saline solution may be purchased over the counter or prepared at home by combining salt with distilled or heated water.

Avoiding Nasal Trauma

Patients should avoid activities that may result in nasal injuries. This includes not blowing your nose hard, avoiding heavy lifting, and staying away from contact sports. If sneezing is inevitable, do so with an open mouth to relieve pressure on the healing nasal tissues.

Keeping Nasal Area Clean

The exterior nasal region must be maintained clean and dry. Gently cleaning the region with a clean, wet towel may aid in hygiene. Patients should not use lotions, ointments, or nasal sprays that have not been recommended by their surgeon.

Monitoring for signs of infection

Watch for indications of infection, such as increasing redness, swelling, discomfort, or foul-smelling discharge. If any of these symptoms are present, the patient should call their doctor immediately. Early action may help avert more serious problems.

Potential Complications And Management

While endoscopic sinus surgery is typically safe, there are certain risks that patients should be aware of. Understanding these issues and how to handle them might help people seek prompt medical care if necessary.

Bleeding

Minor bleeding is normal in the first few days after surgery, but excessive bleeding is the reason for worry. If the bleeding is prolonged or excessive, patients should seek emergency medical assistance. Applying a cold compress to the nose and elevating the head might help control mild bleeding.

Infection

Infections may occur after any operation. Patients should follow their antibiotic course exactly as indicated and practice adequate nose hygiene. If indications of infection appear, such as fever, increasing discomfort, or pus-like discharge, call your healthcare professional immediately.

Nasal obstruction

Some individuals may have nasal obstruction owing to edema or crusting. Regular nasal irrigation may help to avoid this, but in certain situations, the surgeon may need to do small in-office operations to remove obstructive crusts or polyps.

Changes in odor or taste

Temporary changes in smell or taste are frequent after sinus surgery. These normally resolve themselves when the nasal tissues repair. However, if these changes continue, patients should consult with their surgeon at follow-up appointments.

Rehabilitation Exercises And Follow-Up Visits

Rehabilitation and follow-up care are critical aspects of the postoperative period. They promote appropriate healing and assist in restoring normal nasal function.

Breathing exercises

Breathing exercises may help improve nasal airflow and lung capacity. Simple exercises, such as deep breathing, in which patients gently inhale with their nose and expel through their mouth, may be effective. These exercises should be performed in a comfortable setting, gradually increasing in time as comfort permits.

Physical activity

While vigorous activity should be avoided in the beginning, mild physical activities such as walking may be resumed after a few weeks. Patients should listen to their bodies and gradually raise their exercise levels depending on their comfort and their healthcare provider's recommendations.

Follow-up visits

Regular follow-up visits are critical for tracking the healing process. During these appointments, the surgeon will examine the nasal passageways for symptoms of problems, remove crusts, and verify that the sinuses heal correctly. These appointments also allow people to address any issues or symptoms they are experiencing.

Long-Term Care

Even after the first healing phase, continued care is essential. Patients should continue to have frequent nasal irrigations and follow-up visits as indicated by their healthcare physician. Long-term treatment may also include avoiding recognized allergens or irritants that might cause sinus problems.

Patients who follow these postoperative care instructions and keep open contact with their healthcare practitioner may improve their recovery and get the best possible results following endoscopic sinus surgery.

CHAPTER 8:

Advancements In Endoscopic Sinus Surgery

Emerging Technologies

High Definition Endoscopy

High-definition (HD) endoscopy has transformed sinus surgery by allowing surgeons to see more clearly the complicated architecture of the nasal cavity and sinuses. HD endoscopes provide clearer images, enabling more accurate identification of anatomical landmarks and disease alterations. This technique lowers the risk of complications and boosts the success rate of procedures by allowing for more precise dissections and resections.

Image-guided Surgery (IGS)

Image-guided surgery (IGS) systems employ preoperative CT images to generate a 3D map of the patient's sinus architecture.

During surgery, this map is combined with real-time monitoring of surgical tools, giving the physician exact position data. IGS is especially useful in difficult or revision procedures where deformed anatomy may be a barrier. IGS improves the safety and effectiveness of sinus procedures by reducing the chance of inadvertently damaging important tissues such as the optic nerve or brain.

Powered Instruments

The use of powered devices, such as microdebriders and shavers, has greatly enhanced the efficiency and accuracy of tissue removal during endoscopic sinus surgery. These devices enable the controlled removal of polyps and damaged mucosa with little impact on the surrounding tissues. The use of powered equipment has also decreased operational and postoperative recovery times.

Balloon Sinuplasty

Balloon sinuplasty is a minimally invasive procedure that employs a tiny, flexible balloon catheter to widen a clogged sinus ostium. When inflated, the balloon gradually restructures and opens the sinus apertures, restoring normal drainage without requiring tissue excision. Compared to standard surgical approaches, this technique results in less blood, less postoperative discomfort, and quicker recovery durations.

Innovative Surgical Techniques

Draf Procedures

Draf operations, often called frontal sinus drill-out procedures, are sophisticated approaches for treating difficult frontal sinus illnesses. The Draf II and Draf III operations remove the frontal sinus floor and interspinous septum, resulting in a wide shared drainage route.

These treatments are recommended for individuals with persistent frontal sinusitis and provide long-term relief by providing proper drainage and ventilation.

Minimally Invasive Approaches

Recent advances in endoscopic technology and methods have allowed for more minimally invasive sinus surgery procedures. Techniques such as the "swing-door" technique for frontal sinusotomy and the "reverse" Ethmoidectomy for difficult-to-reach locations provide excellent disease care while causing minimum damage to normal structure. These treatments result in reduced postoperative pain and a speedier recovery.

Use of Biological Adjuncts

Biological adjuncts, such as drug-eluting stents and topical corticosteroid treatments, are increasingly being used to improve sinus surgery results. Drug-eluting stents provide medicine directly to the surgery site, decreasing inflammation and aiding recovery. Furthermore, topical corticosteroids may help preserve sinus patency and prevent disease recurrence after surgery.

Office-Based Procedures

Endoscopic technology has advanced to the point that many sinus treatments may now be done in the office under local anesthetic. Office-based operations, such as balloon sinuplasty and small polypectomies, are more convenient, less expensive, and have faster recovery periods than typical operating room surgery. Patients gain from the reduction in the requirement for general anesthesia and its accompanying hazards.

Future Directions For Sinus Surgery

Robotics for Sinus Surgery

Robotic-assisted surgery is a growing area that has the potential to improve accuracy and control in endoscopic sinus treatments.

Robotic devices may improve surgeons' dexterity and stability, enabling them to execute difficult tasks with ease. The use of robots in sinus surgery is predicted to enhance results and broaden the scope of disorders that may be treated endoscopically.

Regenerative Medicine

Regenerative medicine provides intriguing treatment options for chronic sinus illness. Tissue engineering and stem cell treatment are techniques aimed at restoring normal sinus mucosa and function. Research is now underway to find ways to repair damaged tissues and improve the long-term consequences of sinus surgery.

Augmented Reality (AR)

Augmented reality (AR) is being investigated as a technique for improving surgical vision and navigation. AR overlays digital information onto the surgeon's field of vision, allowing enabling real-time guidance during surgeries. This technique may increase the precision of anatomical structures and diseases, resulting in more accurate and successful procedures.

CHAPTER 9

Patient Education And Communication

Educating Patients On Their Condition

Before getting into the complexities of endoscopic sinus surgery (ESS), patients must understand their problem completely. This includes detailing the structure of the sinuses, how they work, and how different disorders, such as chronic sinusitis or nasal polyps, might affect their health and quality of life.

Patients should be given simple, jargon-free explanations of their diagnosis, including any imaging results such as CT scans or nasal endoscopic findings. Visual aids, such as anatomical models or diagrams, may help patients understand complicated subjects more readily.

Furthermore, it is critical to address the symptoms they are having and how they connect to their sinus problem. Understanding the precise signs and symptoms allows individuals to better detect when their disease is deteriorating or when they need to seek medical assistance.

Furthermore, teaching patients about the different treatment choices available, including surgical and non-surgical treatments, allows them to make more educated healthcare decisions. This conversation should go over the possible advantages, hazards, and limits of each alternative, enabling patients to consider their options based on their preferences and objectives.

Finally, further education is essential. Patients should be encouraged to ask questions, seek clarification, and remain educated about their illness throughout the treatment process. Providing trustworthy resources, such as credible websites, support groups, or instructional materials, ensures that people can get appropriate information even outside of therapeutic settings.

Communicating The Risks And Benefits Of Surgery

When choosing endoscopic sinus surgery (ESS), patients should have a thorough grasp of both the risks and advantages of the treatment. Clear and open communication between healthcare practitioners and patients is critical in this situation.

First and foremost, patients should be educated about the possible advantages of ESS, which include increased sinus drainage, decreased frequency and severity of sinus infections, relief of symptoms such as nasal congestion or face discomfort, and improved overall quality of life. By emphasizing these possible positive outcomes, patients might have a greater understanding of how surgery can affect their health and well-being.

It is equally vital to address the possible hazards and problems of ESS. These may include, but are not limited to, bleeding, infection, injury to adjacent tissues such as the eyes or brain, changes in sense of smell or taste, and the necessity for future surgery. While these dangers are uncommon, patients should be aware of them so that they may make educated treatment choices.

In addition to presenting the overall dangers and advantages of ESS, it is critical to tailor this information depending on each patient's unique circumstances. Overall health, medical history, intensity of symptoms, and treatment objectives may all have an impact on surgical results. Tailoring the talk to these particular issues ensures that patients understand what to anticipate before, during, and after the treatment.

Finally, open communication builds confidence between patients and healthcare professionals, allowing them to actively engage in treatment choices and take control of their health.

Addressing Patients' Concerns And Expectations

Endoscopic sinus surgery (ESS) may cause patients to have a variety of anxieties and expectations, ranging from dread of the unknown to hope of symptom alleviation. Addressing these issues and managing expectations successfully is critical to achieving a happy surgery experience and optimum results.

One major worry among ESS patients is the possibility of experiencing pain or discomfort during the process. It is critical to reassure patients that current surgical procedures, such as the use of local or general anesthetic, reduce discomfort during the procedure itself. Furthermore, post-operative discomfort may usually be efficiently controlled with medication and other supportive treatments such as nasal irrigation or humidification.

Another common worry expressed by patients is the risk of complications or unpleasant events after surgery. Patients may make educated treatment choices by receiving comprehensive information regarding the risks and advantages of ESS, while also being aware that problems, albeit uncommon, are possible. Emphasizing the necessity of post-operative care, follow-up visits, and taking prescribed medicines might help to alleviate these fears.

Managing patient expectations is just as crucial in the setting of ESS. While the surgery may provide considerable symptom relief and enhance the quality of life for many patients, it is important to note that individual results may differ. The severity of the underlying sinus condition, anatomical variances, and general health all have an impact on the surgery's outcome and recovery time. Setting reasonable expectations for the expected outcomes and recovery process allows patients to approach surgery with readiness and confidence.

Open and honest communication is critical in resolving patient concerns and matching expectations throughout the surgical process. Encouraging patients to express their concerns, anxieties, and preferences develops a collaborative connection between healthcare professionals and patients, which leads to a happy surgery experience and optimum results.

Resources For Ongoing Support And Information

Endoscopic sinus surgery (ESS) is a journey that continues beyond the operating room, and patients benefit immensely from continued care and information throughout and after their recovery. Providing patients with materials to help them traverse this path allows them to actively engage in their treatment and make educated health choices.

Patients undergoing ESS benefit from having access to educational resources that reinforce essential themes presented during treatment visits. These materials may include booklets, brochures, or online resources that include themes such as pre-operative preparation, what to anticipate during surgery, post-operative care instructions, and frequently asked questions. By providing these materials in a variety of forms, patients may evaluate information at their speed and go back to it as required.

In addition to instructional resources, support groups may be quite beneficial for individuals undergoing ESS. Connecting with individuals who have had similar surgeries helps patients to share their experiences, discuss advice for managing symptoms and recovery, and provide emotional support to one another. Support groups, whether in person or online, provide a feeling of connection and understanding, which may significantly improve the patient experience.

Furthermore, regular contact with healthcare professionals is critical to ensure that patients feel supported throughout their healing process. Encouraging patients to contact them with any questions, concerns, or updates enables healthcare practitioners to give tailored assistance and resolve any difficulties that occur. Regular follow-up sessions also allow us to evaluate progress, analyze results, and make any required changes to the treatment plan.

Finally, providing patients with options for continuous support and knowledge enables them to actively participate in their recovery and long-term sinus health. Healthcare practitioners may help patients transition smoothly and successfully from surgery to long-term wellness by providing them with the necessary information and support.

CHAPTER 10
Lifestyle Changes And Long-Term Management

Importance Of Lifestyle Changes

Lifestyle changes are critical for successfully controlling sinus symptoms. While medical treatments such as drugs and procedures are necessary, making some lifestyle modifications may improve their efficacy and help overall sinus health.

One of the most significant reasons for making lifestyle modifications is that they may assist address the underlying causes or triggers of sinus issues. For example, avoiding environmental allergens like pollen, dust, and pet dander might minimize the frequency and severity of sinus symptoms in those who are prone to allergic rhinitis.

Similarly, stopping smoking may boost sinus health by lowering inflammation and irritation in the nasal passages.

Furthermore, lifestyle changes may supplement medical therapies by enhancing general health. A balanced diet rich in fruits, vegetables, and whole grains contains critical nutrients that promote immune function and lower inflammation, which may help those with chronic sinusitis. Regular exercise may help increase immune function and circulation, assisting in the removal of mucus from the sinuses.

Furthermore, lifestyle adjustments may help people manage stress, which is known to worsen sinus problems. Deep breathing, meditation, and yoga are examples of relaxation exercises that may help decrease stress and enhance a feeling of well-being, perhaps leading to fewer sinus flare-ups.

General, lifestyle adjustments are important for controlling sinus disorders since they address both the underlying reasons and the individual's general health. Individuals who practice healthy behaviors may lessen their dependency on drugs, lower the frequency and severity of sinus problems, and enhance their overall quality of life.

Strategies To Prevent Sinus Issues

Preventing sinus problems entails employing a variety of techniques aimed at decreasing exposure to triggers while maintaining optimum sinus health. These techniques include environmental, nutritional, and behavioral adjustments that may reduce the likelihood of sinusitis and other sinus-related issues.

One of the most effective prophylactic methods is to avoid recognized allergies and irritants. This includes reducing exposure to airborne allergens like pollen, dust mites, and mold by utilizing air purifiers, cleaning interior areas regularly, and closing windows during peak pollen seasons. Similarly, limiting your exposure to cigarette smoke, air pollution, and other environmental toxins may help reduce sinus inflammation and irritation.

Maintaining excellent hygiene habits is also important for avoiding sinus problems. This involves often washing your hands to avoid the transmission of viruses and bacteria that may cause sinus infections. A saline nasal rinse or spray may help cleanse the nasal passages of mucus and allergens, lowering the risk of sinus congestion and infection.

Dietary choices might also affect nasal health. A diet high in anti-inflammatory foods such fruits, vegetables, and whole grains and omega-3 fatty acids may help decrease nasal inflammation and improve immunological function. Furthermore, keeping hydrated by consuming enough of water might help thin mucus discharges, making them simpler to remove from the sinuses.

Maintaining a healthy lifestyle, which includes regular exercise, proper sleep, and stress management, may also help to avoid sinus problems. Exercise enhances circulation and immunological function, and appropriate sleep enables the body to repair and renew tissues, including those in the sinuses. Stress management practices such as deep breathing, meditation, and yoga may help decrease inflammation and improve general well-being.

Individuals who follow these preventative practices may lower their chance of acquiring sinus problems and maintain excellent sinus health.

Long-Term Treatment Of Chronic Sinusitis

Chronic sinusitis requires long-term therapy that includes a multidimensional strategy aimed at managing symptoms, avoiding flare-ups, and improving the overall quality of life for those suffering from the illness.

While medical treatments like drugs and surgery may be required, lifestyle changes and continued self-care are also important aspects of long-term management.

One of the key aims of long-term treatment is to reduce inflammation and infection in the sinuses. Nasal corticosteroids, antibiotics, and antihistamines are often used to decrease inflammation, remove infection, and treat symptoms such as congestion, face discomfort, and nasal discharge. Individuals with allergic rhinitis may benefit from immunotherapy to desensitize their immune systems to particular allergens.

In addition to medicine, daily nasal irrigation with saline solution may aid in the removal of mucus and allergens from the nasal passages, decreasing congestion and infection. This may be accomplished using a squeeze bottle, neti pot, or nasal irrigation equipment, with correct cleanliness and technique to reduce the risk of problems.

When medicinal therapies fail or symptoms are severe, surgery may be required to enhance sinus drainage and ventilation. Endoscopic sinus surgery is a minimally invasive treatment that is carried out via the nostrils utilizing a thin, flexible scope equipped with a camera and surgical equipment. This enables the exact excision of diseased tissue, expansion of sinus apertures, and correction of anatomical defects that cause sinusitis.

Surgery, on the other hand, is often seen as a last option and is usually reserved for those who have severe or recurring chronic sinusitis that has not responded to previous therapies. Following surgery, long-term care may include frequent follow-up meetings with an ear, nose, and throat (ENT) specialist, continuous nasal irrigation, and preventative measures to limit the chance of recurrence.

In addition to medicinal therapies, lifestyle changes are critical for the long-term management of chronic sinusitis. This involves avoiding recognized triggers like allergies and irritants, practicing excellent hygiene, and leading a healthy lifestyle that includes regular exercise, enough sleep, and stress management skills.

Chronic sinusitis patients may successfully control their disease and improve their quality of life over time by combining medical therapies with lifestyle changes and continued self-care.

Integrative Approaches To Sinus Health

Integrative methods for sinus health combine traditional medical treatments with complementary and alternative therapies to address the root causes of sinus problems and enhance general well-being. These techniques acknowledge the interdependence of the body's systems and seek to treat the whole person rather than simply the symptoms of sinusitis.

One of the cornerstones of integrative medicine is customized therapy, which takes into consideration each person's unique health history, symptoms, and preferences. This may include a mix of traditional medical treatments such as drugs and surgery, as well as alternative therapies including acupuncture, chiropractic therapy, herbal supplements, and nutritional counseling.

Acupuncture, a traditional Chinese medical treatment that involves inserting small needles into particular sites on the body, has been demonstrated to alleviate sinus symptoms like congestion, discomfort, and inflammation. Similarly, chiropractic adjustments may assist improve spinal alignment and nerve function, perhaps leading to greater nasal drainage and ventilation.

Integrative methods for sinus health often include the use of herbal remedies and dietary adjustments. Natural treatments like bromelain, quercetin, and butterbur have anti-inflammatory and immune-modulating characteristics that may help decrease sinus inflammation and alleviate symptoms. Furthermore, dietary changes, such as avoiding dairy and gluten, which are major triggers for certain people, may help relieve sinus problems.

Meditation, biofeedback, and guided imagery are all examples of mind-body therapies that may help manage stress and promote relaxation, potentially reducing inflammation and improving sinus health. These strategies may be used alone or as part of a larger integrated therapy strategy.

While integrative methods for sinus health may not be appropriate for everyone, they do provide additional choices for those looking for alternatives or supplements to traditional medical therapies. Integrative treatments may help people obtain long-term relief and a higher quality of life by treating the root causes of sinus problems and boosting overall well-being.

Conclusion

In conclusion, knowing endoscopic sinus surgery (ESS) is critical for patients, clinicians, and medical workers. This detailed guide has shed light on the subtle nuances of ESS, from its historical origins to its current implementations. We've set out to demystify this complex surgical process by investigating the architecture of the sinuses, the pathophysiology of sinusitis, and advances in endoscopic procedures.

ESS has transformed the treatment of chronic rhinosinusitis and other sinus-related illnesses, providing patients with a less invasive approach that has lower morbidity and quicker recovery periods than standard open operations. Endoscopes allow surgeons to see and treat sick tissue directly in the sinuses, resulting in better results and patient satisfaction.

Patient selection and preoperative assessment are critical to the effectiveness of ESS. The surgical approach is guided by a thorough evaluation of symptoms, imaging tests, and functional testing, resulting in tailored therapy and the best results. Furthermore, recognizing the possible risks and problems of ESS allows patients and healthcare professionals to make more educated choices and reduce the likelihood of adverse outcomes.

Postoperative care is critical to the healing phase after ESS. Close monitoring, adherence to recommended drugs, and timely follow-up sessions are critical components of a positive result. Patients should be informed on good nasal hygiene and lifestyle changes to reduce the chance of illness recurrence while maximizing long-term benefits.

As with any surgical intervention, continued research and innovation drive progress in ESS, broadening treatment choices and improving surgical procedures. Collaboration among otolaryngologists, allergists, immunologists, and other experts promotes a multidisciplinary approach to sinus treatment, therefore enhancing patient management and quality of life.

The full guide to understanding endoscopic sinus surgery is an invaluable resource for patients, caregivers, and healthcare professionals navigating the complexity of sinus illness and its treatment. By increasing information, understanding, and teamwork, we can continue to refine and improve sinus care delivery, eventually resulting in better results and improved patient well-being.

THE END

www.ingramcontent.com/pod-product-compliance
Lightning Source LLC
Chambersburg PA
CBHW071835210526
45479CB00001B/148